BRAIN STORMING

The Serper Method of Brain Recovery, Regrowth, and Vitality

How to rehabilitate your brain
after a stroke or other cerebral trauma.

How to keep your brain alive
during the early stages of Alzheimer's disease and other age-related memory losses.

© 2000 by Lynn Lazarus Serper, Ed.D.
All rights reserved.
ISBN 0-9678718-0-8

Published by
Brain Enhancement Services, Inc.
770 Boylston Street, Suite 17-I
Boston, MA 02199
800-240-3778
E-Mail: brainsharp@aol.com
www.brainenhance.com

Dedication

This book is dedicated to my children and their spouses:
Susie and Howard, Jay and Robyn, and Layne and Kurt.
And to my grandchildren:
Allison, Max and Harrison, Madeline and Jake, and Henry.

…for the joy and energy they bring to my life.

TABLE OF CONTENTS

INTRODUCTION/1

MY STORY/7

WHO AM I?/WHO ARE YOU?/19

SUDDENLY A CAREGIVER/23

THE ROLE OF ADULT CHILDREN/31

THE ROLE OF GRANDCHILDREN/35

HOW FRIENDS CAN HELP/39

SEEKING EMOTIONAL SUPPORT/43

THE RESEARCH/47

THE PROGRAM/53

USING THE PROGRAM WITH PEOPLE IN
EARLY STAGES OF ALZHEIMER'S DISEASE/61

HOW THE PROGRAM WORKS/71

HOW TO USE THE SERPER METHOD FOR YOUR OWN
BRAIN RECOVERY, REGROWTH, AND VITALITY/75

APPENDIX A:
THE SERPER METHOD WORKBOOK (SAMPLE PAGES)/123

APPENDIX B:
SELF-HELP BOOKS FOR CAREGIVERS/129

APPENDIX C:
ORDER FORMS/133

ACKNOWLEDGEMENTS

I want to thank my "recovery team" of professionals: Robin Goldberg, Mary Packard, Ruona Bertaccini, Albyn Davis, Grace Craig, Rockie Blunt, Aviva Wynn, Sidney Smith, and Randall Long.

I want to thank my "recovery team" of friends: Shirley and Bob Siff, Nathan Cohen, Marilyn Perlman, Renee, Hal, Lissa, Marlyse, and Beth Rudnick, Barbara Burwick, Beth Coolidge, Priscilla and Kenny Jacobson, Harlee Chandler, Carolyn Salk, Sylvia Strauss, and Ruth Baum.

I want to thank Geoff Harvey, my colleague and co-creator of Brain Enhancement Services, Inc., and his son, Peter Harvey, for keeping us organized.

I also want to thank all of the people who share in my belief that my program for brain recovery, regrowth, and vitality really does work.

Finally, this may be "my" story and "my" program, but I never would have had the time for it to become "my" book, were it not for my collaborator, Dr. Dale Koppel.

Introduction

I had thought about calling this book, "Don't Believe What Your Doctors Tell You: You CAN Restore Your Brain Power." As you read my story and use my program, you'll see why it would have been an excellent title.

Had I let my family follow doctors' orders, I wouldn't have had the opportunity to write this book either. The doctors held out little hope for my mental recovery. They rarely do in these cases. The damage done to my brain had rendered me unable to write, count, or comprehend written or spoken information. I suffered from short-term memory loss and limited vocabulary

Introduction

retrieval. My speech was slow, halting, and, even worse, confused. I couldn't find the words to express my thoughts.

This book is literally a labor of blood, sweat, tears, and love. It's not a book that I ever thought I'd write. After all, I never thought I'd become a stroke victim at age 48. Or ever, for that matter.

So, how did this book come to be?

Perhaps I've always been the curious type, always wondering why something works and why something else doesn't. Maybe that's what intrigued me most as a teacher for 11 years. Maybe that's what challenged me to teach children with learning disabilities, and what motivated me to enter into a doctoral program at the University of Massachusetts at Amherst to further understand cognitive development – how people think and how they learn.

And then…

Introduction

Before I finished my doctoral work, a ruptured aneurysm, followed by a cerebral stroke, reduced me to the learning-disabled child I had once taught.

Five years after my stroke, at age 53, I became the stroke survivor who wanted to teach again. This time, though, I would teach others who were still trapped in the victim stage, the people who were experiencing the same feelings of hopelessness that I had experienced.

I spent four years developing The Serper Method of Brain Recovery, Regrowth, and Vitality as a user-friendly brain therapy program. I can now offer it to others, who need it in the same way I needed it, through Brain Enhancement Services, Inc., the company I established to work with individuals, hospitals, assisted living facilities, and other agencies. Some of my clients like to call me their personal brain trainer.

Now, through this book and additional workbooks and activities, I am able to provide an opportunity for others to know that recovery is possible and that they can incorporate The Serper Method of Brain Recovery, Regrowth, and Vitality into their personal lives.

I suppose I didn't need to have a stroke in order to develop the curriculum that is the basis for my brain rehabilitation program. After all, I had a background in education; I was an excellent developer of curriculum. But, had I not had the stroke, I would have never known the crying need for someone to put together a self-rehabilitation program that would address the issues of brain recovery and regrowth.

This is a book and a program that I wish I had had when I was fighting to regain my cerebral functioning.

In the area of stroke rehabilitation, the primary focus has most often been on the physical. Maybe that's because brain research is still a new, albeit growing, field. After all, the brain isn't something you can look at, or physically move around, like an arm or a leg. And even though someone may never walk again, may always be confined to a wheelchair, or worse, a bed, there's at least an effort to try to do something about the physical limitations.

You will also read how my program has helped people who are in the early stages of Alzheimer's disease.

If you are a caregiver, I hope that you will share or read portions of this book to the person you are caring for, and care about. I hope that my personal story will serve as an inspiration.

My own brain rehabilitation took five years and a lot of hard work. It also took a willingness – and a determination – to work hard.

Of course, I wish that I had never had the stroke, never had my survival skills tested. Still, I must say that it made me feel incredible when my daughter, Layne, told me, "You're the old you, only a better version because you now know you can accomplish anything."

Recently, my nine-year-old granddaughter, Allison, and I were having dinner together, and I told her that I had just finished a book.

(You will read in my chapter, "The Role of Grandchildren," how important Allison actually was to my recovery.)

"What is it about?" she asked me.

"It's about me, and how I got sick and better, and how I can help other people," I replied.

And with all the naive enthusiasm and seriousness only an adorable (and I write that with total objectivity!) nine-year-old can exude, she said, "Now, that's a book I have to read."

My Story

It really was a dark and stormy night, the night of October 10, 1990, when this story begins. So dark and stormy, in fact, that my plane from New York City to Worcester, Massachusetts, where I lived, had to land in Boston – an hour's van ride away from home.

Under other circumstances, I probably wouldn't have minded – so much. But, on this particular night, I was feeling extraordinarily tired. I had been visiting my father, and it had been a difficult week.

At age 48, I was experiencing the stress of being a member of the sandwich generation. My father was 89 years old and living alone. A couple of months earlier, he had suffered a heart attack. He refused to move to New England, and I would not move to New York. We agreed that, as his designated caregiver, I would spend a week each month with him.

There was a lot going on for me at the time. I had separated from my husband 10 months earlier and was trying to complete my doctoral dissertation in Human Cognitive Development. I was cultivating a new romance and helping my oldest daughter plan her June wedding. I was also finding time to spend with my son and daughter-in-law's new baby – my first grandchild. It still makes me tired just thinking about it.

As I sat waiting for the van to take me home, I suddenly felt an odd pain over my right eye. It moved in slowly, almost imperceptibly. At first, it felt like a gentle wave spreading over sand. Then, the wave started pounding, the intensity and pain so great, my entire head began to throb.

I convinced myself that resting against the back seat of the van, breathing deeply and thinking lovely thoughts, would calm the storm in my head by the time I reached home. But instead, it worsened.

I remember getting out of the van and walking through my back door into the kitchen. Then, nothing.

My son, Jay, tells me that he found me in my bedroom – in bed, an overturned telephone on the floor, an unopened bottle of Bufferin in my hand. But that wasn't until almost 24 hours later. He tells me that my eyes were open and that I looked right at him. He knew I wanted to talk to him, but I couldn't. He tells me I looked like a person stuck inside my own body. I don't remember any of it.

The doctors tell me that I had had a ruptured brain aneurysm; two bubbles in an artery in my head had ruptured, and surgery was required.

Everything probably would have been fine except that the day after surgery, I suffered a cerebral stroke and remained in a semi-coma for three weeks.

Isn't it strange how the brain works? I mean, there I was opening my eyes for the first time in more than three weeks. And I looked around the room and thought, "I am in a hospital; I have had a stroke; and now I have aphasia." (Aphasia, a word that I had learned about as a learning disabilities teacher, is the inability to use, remember, or comprehend the spoken or written word.)

I even knew the extent of the damage that I had suffered.

"I cannot read; I cannot count; I cannot find the words I need to express what I'm thinking, so of course I cannot say any of this out loud," I said to myself.

I could also tell that the stroke had left me with

a serious weakness that encompassed the entire right side of my body, but luckily I wasn't paralyzed.

I was lying in my hospital bed when the door opened. It was my friend, Nate Cohen, checking in on me.

Now, tell me. How lucky can a person be having a friend who is not only a doctor, but also an orthopedic surgeon with a broad knowledge of rehabilitative medicine?

He stood at the foot of my bed, looked me straight in the eye, and told me, "I looked at your records, and you're going to get your language and thinking skills back. It's going to take a long time and a lot of hard work, but you will get all of your skills back."

Oh, how I clung to those words. Truly, they became the mantra of my recovery.

It wasn't until years later that I learned that there wasn't an ounce of truth to it. He was trying to give me hope. And it worked.

But, at the time, he was the only one who even pretended. And the only one who recommended rehabilitation centers; ones that considered language therapy as important as physical therapy.

The doctors told my family to take me home and provide me with "a lot of love and long-term care." Hire people who would bathe me, dress me, cook for me, get me into a wheelchair, and sit me in front of the television.

But the opportunity to attend and participate in two rehabilitation centers – and the belief that I would improve – started me on the road to recovery.

How to describe the next five years?

I spent three-and-half months at two rehabilitation centers: The first two months at the Rusk Institute of Rehabilitation in New York City and, then, six weeks at the Communication Disorders Clinic at the University of Michigan in Ann Arbor.

My Story

The Rusk Institute of Rehabilitation and the Communication Disorders Clinic at the University of Michigan both offered comprehensive cognitive rehabilitation. Typically, rehabilitation centers believe that if the physical body is exercised, it will be restored, or at least regain some of its strength. But if the brain is damaged, many feel that there isn't much to be gained from cognitive and memory exercises, even though they're designed to restore cerebral functioning, or at least regain some of its strength.

I was going to prove that theory wrong. Those words – "You will get your skills back, but it will require a lot of work" – absolutely consumed me. All I wanted to do was work. And when it wasn't forthcoming, I demanded it – plaintively – in two- or three-word sentences: "More work." "I need homework." "I have to (recover)." Of course, I couldn't retrieve the words from my brain to describe the type of work I wanted; I had to just be grateful for what I was given.

I became a clock-watcher. I was supposed to

have physical therapy at 9 a.m., and if it was 9:02 a.m., and the physical therapist had not started working with me, I went into a panic. I saw it as being robbed of two minutes of opportunity to recover.

The only emotion I experienced was anger, anger if someone didn't have something for me to do all the time. Otherwise, I was devoid of feelings. I never felt scared; I never felt sad. I was consumed by determination.

About six weeks after I started my rehabilitation at Rusk, I rolled myself into the occupational therapy room and noticed an old Royal typewriter. I could think in my head, and I could write in my head, and suddenly I had this idea that my fingers could talk for me.

Finally, a way to communicate. I was so excited at the prospect. So, I wheeled myself over to the table and put my fingers on the keys and waited for the thoughts to reach my finger tips. Nothing. I started to push the keys so frantically that they all stuck to the paper. When I got them back in place, I looked at the page. Jibberish.

And then I started to cry. For the first time since I had had my stroke, I cried. Boy, did I cry. It was as though someone had opened the flood gates. I couldn't stop. I cried through the rest of my rehab therapy sessions that day, and when I finally got to my room, I was so exhausted, I couldn't even do my coveted homework.

At the end of two months, I could walk on my own, and express more thoughts, albeit still in a slow and halting way. I could generally let my needs be known, but only through short, simple statements. Oh yes, I could also count. You see, I had become absolutely obsessed with teaching myself how to count again. So, when I had to practice walking, I counted my steps. When I was put on a stationary bicycle, I counted the pedal strokes.

"One, two… two… two."

At first, I couldn't even figure out what came next. "Keep counting," the voice in my head would say. "You can do it. One, two… two… two."

As a teacher, I always believed that my students would either live up to – or down to – my expectations. That's why I always set high expectations for them. It's absolutely criminal when I think about how health care professionals set such low expectations for people who have suffered strokes. And how quick they are to use the word, "plateau," as in, one's recovery has reached a plateau.

Doctors typically point to a three- to six-month "window of opportunity." (It takes about three months for the swelling of the brain to go down after a stroke.) But even at my six-month "anniversary," I couldn't possibly have been able to function on my own. I needed a lot more time to reach that so-called "plateau."

As far as I'm concerned, the only time you reach your plateau is when you give up on yourself. Unfortunately, that's easy to do. That's why it's so important to find someone who will be passionate with you on your behalf.

When I look back, I realize that the people who made the biggest difference in my life were those people who believed in me. (That doesn't necessarily mean that they always genuinely believed that I was going to get better, but at least they made me believe that they believed I was going to get better.) And, when they sat down to work with me, they did so with a purpose and a goal – to get me better. ME. They made me feel that we were a team and – this is really key, too – that they liked being with me, that they weren't just "doing a job." Those were the people who tried to do things with me that tapped into my particular interests. That made me feel as though I was an individual. These days, when I am invited to speak to college students who are studying to become future speech therapists, this is what I tell them. And what I'm telling you – again – is, find someone who will be passionate on your behalf.

Who Am I? / Who Are You?

Society often writes off stroke victims because they're not who they once were. As a result, stroke victims write themselves off – for the same reason. They're not the person they once were. Worse, they don't know how to get that person back.

The painful reality is that they will never get that same person back. But often – over time – a better person will emerge.

Sometimes, when I think back to the person I used to be, I wonder whether I really listened to others, or whether I was more interested in telling them about myself. After my stroke, I had to become a listener – if I ever wanted to be in social situations again. And, as far as I'm concerned, getting back into social situations (and that includes being able to talk on the phone and leave messages on answering machines) is essential in order to get from stroke victim to stroke survivor.

In order to get back into social situations, with the help of language therapists, I practiced asking socially-appropriate (as in, "small-talk") questions; you know, the "who, what, where, why, how, when" questions. I practiced nodding my head when others spoke even though, at the time, what they were saying was much too complicated for me to understand. After awhile, I trained myself to hold onto the last thing a person said, so that I could ask another question (related to what they had just said) before they had a chance to ask me a question. If they did ask me a question, I practiced ways to avoid answering them. How? By saying things like, "I'll tell you later."

Sometimes, I really wanted to answer a question, and I'd find myself stumbling for words. I learned how to say, "Oh, never mind," and then ask another question as quickly as I could. Try it sometime. You'll probably be amazed to see how well it works – with anyone. When it comes right down to it, people would much rather talk about themselves than about you.

Suddenly a Caregiver

So far, I have written primarily about myself. Now, this chapter focuses on the caregiver – a spouse, a friend, a partner, a relative.

The harsh reality is that in an instant – with no warning, no time to prepare – you become a caregiver. Your own life changes as abruptly as the person's who has suffered the trauma. You are no longer the person you once were, nor do you have the relationship you once had. Your role has changed, too. Suddenly, as caregiver, you must be teacher, therapist, advocate, stand-up comedian, chief liar ("You will recover…"), and parent. The papa (or mama) bear has become the baby bear.

It's as simple – and complicated – as that.

Still, whenever possible, you want to try to replicate the life you had before. It requires some creativity on your part – and seeing the proverbial glass half full, not half empty. (Don't ever underestimate the importance of a positive attitude.)

How can you replicate your previous life together? Here are some examples:

If the two of you traveled a lot before, but can't now, watch travel videos instead. Look through travel magazines together. Take out the photos of the trips you took. Talk about them.

Did you find humor in your life before? If you can't find humor in your present situation, find it elsewhere. Read the humorous stories and columns in Reader's Digest. Watch comedy videos. Re-visit those movies that used to make the two of you laugh.

It's a matter of redefining who you are now – and the scope of your new possibilities. You are the only one who can do that. No one else can tell you what to do – and if they try, and it doesn't fit into your design, don't listen. This is the time to listen to your inner voice. This is the time to get your antennae up and running, your radar fine-tuned.

You are going to have to make decisions on your loved one's behalf, based not only on information you receive (solicited or unsolicited), but also on what your "gut" tells you. And if your gut tells you that the system is not providing for your situation, you need to do the "standing up for." Investigate. Research. (If you don't have one already, buy a computer; take an Internet course.) Advocate. Write letters – to legislators, to editors. Network.

Finding and/or creating an inner physical, mental, and emotional strength is your first step. Imagine that you have been asked to build a house from the ground up. You need to start with the foundation. If the foundation is solid, everything else will follow. Easy to say, right? Harder to do. This is the challenge.

Of course, you're going to grieve. You have lost

the person you once knew, and you probably won't get him, or her, back in the old form. But there is/will be a new form. Elements of it may even be better.

"He's not so arrogant anymore," the spouse of one of my clients once told me. "I see a much softer side."

(I think I'm still a better listener than I was before I had my stroke.)

Your grieving is a reality, but it can – and should – be directed toward creating new opportunities, and ultimately coming up with successful strategies.

Ultimately, I had to become my own caregiver. In thinking back over that period of time, I realize that much of what I did for myself was in my role as caregiver; much of what I did was as the stroke survivor. Sometimes, the two were interconnected.

I felt that I had to turn my recovery into a business. Call it "Getting Healthy, Inc." As caregiver, I was the CEO. If you've retired from whatever your previous job was (including parenting), then think of it this way: You have to come out of retirement;

get back on the work train.

For what may have been the first time in my life, I had to start thinking "outside the box." I had to start seeking alternative outlets. I really don't think that in my "past life," for example, I would have ever considered The Feldenkrais Method as a way to rehabilitate myself physically.

I was fortunate that Aviva Wynn, a certified Feldenkrais instructor, taught me about mind-body movement (The Feldenkrais Method), and now, I recommend it as part of the recovery plan for my clients who need to improve their flexibility and ease of movement. Because the exercises are designed to enhance the communication between the brain and the body, it essentially becomes a brainstorming supplement to my program. I also recommend Feldenkrais for many caregivers of my clients – for stress reduction. In that way, it also offers an opportunity for caregiver and survivor to share a new experience together.

Probably one of the biggest challenges caregivers will face is knowing how much to do, and when to step back. If you raised a child, you can probably remember the milestones, like her first step. And you can probably remember how hard it was to hold back, to let her fall, pick herself up, take a step, fall again. That's what caring for a stroke survivor is all about.

Here's an example:

I returned home from Michigan five months after that dark and stormy night in October. Nate Cohen, my doctor-friend, agreed to help me get settled. Of course, the cupboards and refrigerator were bare, so we made a shopping list. I put it in my handbag, and we headed for the supermarket. Of course, I expected that Nate would take care of everything. After all, I could barely talk; I was easily confused; and my memory was still significantly impaired.

We found a cart; I took the list out of my handbag and started looking at it. When I turned around, Nate was gone. He just disappeared.

I felt totally abandoned and scared and angry. The first thing I did was cry. And cry. Then, suddenly, my anger took over. How could a friend desert me like this, I wondered. Who needs friends like this, I said to myself. As had happened before, my anger and frustration turned into determination. If you're going to survive, that voice in my head was saying, you better learn how to shop.

I have no idea how long it took, but I do know it took a very long time. I walked up and down each aisle, trying desperately to match what was on the shelves with what was on the list. Even figuring out how to find the check-out line was a challenge, but when I finally got to the cashier, there was Nate. He looked into my cart filled with food, and then he looked at me and smiled.

I now know why he did what he did. No bird learns to fly if the mother bird keeps bringing the worm to the nest. So, the moral of this example is:

Don't be afraid to turn over responsibilities to your loved one, even though it requires an inordinate amount of patience and perseverance –

and trepidation. The more your loved one participates in the tasks of daily living, working, and interacting, the more skills will be stimulated to return.

Here's something else that you need to keep in mind. Caregivers need care, too. You have to take the time to be good to yourself – without guilt. Again, you're going to need to be creative. For example, if you can't find a support group to join, start one of your own. You'd be surprised at how many other people are out there in a similar situation. You'll find a list of self-help books that I recommend to caregivers in Appendix B.

Sure, there are days when you'll feel ready to give up. Acknowledge that; then let it go. You have to re-define, re-plan, re-create, and re-cover. And please don't ever forget that the core of all healing comes from hope.

The Role of Adult Children

I think – no, I know – it must have been extremely difficult for my three children.

They were in their 20s when this happened. They say that they can still remember how shocked, saddened, and scared they were when they came to the hospital and not only saw me unconscious, but also were told how bad the prognosis was. They weren't prepared for that. After all, they were at that age of invincibility.

They agree that they never thought something like this could happen. Nothing like this had ever happened in our family before.

On the one hand, the more they learned and

The Role of Adult Children

understood, the more comfortable they felt; on the other hand, the more they learned and understood, the more scared they became.

The hardest part for my children was my initial inability to even recognize my youngest daughter, Layne, or my son, Jay, or my oldest daughter, Susie – my own three children! On a "good" day, I might be able to recognize one, but not the others.

But through it all, the three of them never lost their sense of humor.

They once told me, "When you'd recognize only one of us, that person would say, 'See, she loves me more.' But, in reality, we were absolutely devastated."

All of my children remember how I lost my sense of humor (temporarily), how I couldn't follow what they were trying to say to me, and how they couldn't follow what I was trying to say to them. They remember how oversensitive and insecure I could be (and with very good reason).

"It was so hard to watch you struggle," Layne recalls. "And then, as if you suddenly adjusted to the change, you reached a place where you were O.K. with it."

What she didn't realize was that it was my children's support that added to my strength to move forward.

I remember how patient they were with me, and how they helped me in subtle, but essential, ways.

For example, it was because of Susie that I could look into the mirror again. Susie lived in New York and visited me every day while I was at Rusk. Half my head had been shaved during surgery, and the other half hung to my shoulders. I was too vain to look in the mirror, but still too confused to know what to ask for.

One day, Susie suggested that we have "a beauty experience." The next day, she arrived with her hairdresser. And that's how my hair got styled.

Susie admitted that she so desperately wanted to jump in and finish my sentences for me because she could see how I was struggling, how hard it was for me to find the words. But she instinctively knew that if she had, I never would have had to do it myself. And she was right.

Jay says that he could tell that inside I knew everything I wanted to say, so he waited until I got a sentence out.

My children listened to what I had to say. They assumed their caregiver roles graciously, and always treated me with dignity.

In fact, when I completed my doctoral dissertation – in 1995 – I dedicated it to them.

"To my children," I wrote. "For their support, for their love, and because they never let me forget that I was their mother."

The Role of Grandchildren

Grandchildren (if you don't have any of your own, borrow your friends' or neighbors'!) provide respite, emotional strength, and companionship. They also provide the opportunity to play the kinds of games and do the kinds of activities a stroke survivor needs for brain stimulation and redevelopment. A grandchild is like having your own play therapist.

Trust me, this is truly a win-win situation because it's a wonderful learning experience for a grandchild, too. The grandchild who reads to the stroke survivor becomes a better reader. The grandchild who listens while the stroke survivor reads becomes a better listener. The grandchild who participates in the recovery of a beloved grandparent becomes a better person. The experience certainly teaches compassion.

Here's another example of a win-win scenario:

A teenage grandson of one of my clients needed to fulfill community-service hours in order to graduate from high school. He worked with my client – his grandmother – using The Serper Method. He received an "A" on the report he had to write at the end of the semester, and his grandmother sat in the front row of his graduation.

My granddaughter, Allison, was two-and-a-half years old when she started spending afternoons with me. She would bring her games and toys, and we would play together for the entire afternoon.

I loved every minute of it – even the bittersweet moments when it would hit me like a ton of bricks: "Boy, am I in bad shape!"

One day, for example, about a year into our afternoon get-togethers had started, Allison brought a picture matching-card game. I remember deciding that we should only take out a few matching cards because after all, she was only three years old; she wouldn't be able to remember more than a few cards. It turned out that she remembered where they all were. And I couldn't remember where any of them were.

She always brought puzzles with her, and she was always a lot faster at putting the pieces together than I was. More "Boy, am I in bad shape" experiences. But they were also my reality checks. Obviously, at the time, my memory and visual perception level was still below a three-year-old's. It made it clear to me at what level my personal curriculum had to begin. And that was the beginning of The Serper Method curriculum, a recognition that the only sensible place to begin is at the beginning.

I went to a toy store and bought puzzles for

three-year-olds. (I practiced when Allison wasn't around.)

Of course, Allison loved being my playmate. Especially in the beginning, she got to win – legitimately. (O.K., so as I improved, I would sometimes 'let' her win.) I think that there were times that she gave me a break because she sensed that it would make me feel better. (It did.) And maybe winning all the time isn't that much fun after all. Even when you're a three-year-old.

How Friends Can Help

I believe that you need to choose one friend who will provide honest, caring feedback. Someone to whom you can say, for example, "How does my speech sound?" And she won't say, "Oh come on, there's nothing wrong with your speech." But instead, she'll say, "It's better; you seem to be using more words." And then, "I know the pace will pick up if you keep working on it."

You also need a circle of friends who can provide an invaluable service. They can keep you in the friendship "loop" and in that way provide you with the opportunity to be where non-contrived language is taking place. (This is in contrast to contrived language which takes place in settings like language therapy sessions.)

My granddaughter may have been my play therapist. My circle of friends were my social therapists.

They were willing to include me in their activities; they were willing to listen to what I was saying, even though they had to wait patiently for me to make my point, to express what I was trying to say. Without that opportunity to practice, I would have simply lost the will to try.

In the beginning, I could only be the listener. But even as the listener, I still felt as though I belonged, as though I was still in the loop of conversation. And this listening process helped me regain my language skills. Robin Goldberg, my language therapist, told me that the more I listened, the more I'd pick up tone, pace, and inflection. And she was right. I became the professional listener.

Now, that's not to say that I wasn't petrified of putting myself in social situations, especially when the time came that I knew that I could no longer be a listener if I wanted to progress.

I never let my friends know how panicked I was every time they invited me out. What really helped me was writing a list of my fears and then discussing them, one-by-one, in sessions with Robin. That provided me with the opportunity to speak and also to re-frame my fears, mostly by coming up with strategies to overcome them. For example, I wasn't able to carry on a conversation, but I could ask questions, listen to the answer, then ask another question.

I remember one of the biggest challenges for me was being invited to a friend's Christmas party. It was 1992, and I absolutely didn't feel ready. Luckily, though, the invitation came a month in advance. I spent every speech and language therapy session practicing the questions I was going to ask. I call them anticipatory scripts. Here are some examples:

"Do you have any children?"

"What do they do?"

"What line of work are you in?"

"What a lovely pin. Where is it from?"

Everybody loved me! And all I had to do was ask them questions about themselves. I smiled and nodded and never interrupted to turn the subject around to me.

At the end of the evening, I practically danced out the door.

"I did it," I exclaimed to myself, as I put my coat on to leave. "I really did it."

To this day, I can feel the adrenaline pumping.

Seeking Emotional Support

I cannot overstate the importance of seeking emotional support from a professional.

It took me about a year to figure that out. Initially, I couldn't see how going into therapy would help. I was crying over my losses, while working as hard as I could to reach that point of recovery that I believed possible. But oh, it was going so slowly. In fact, when I started realizing how slow the pace of progress actually was, there were many days when I could hardly motivate myself – emotionally – to get out of bed in the morning. That's when I realized I needed someone to talk to, someone who could help me regain my emotional energy.

Someone who has suffered a cerebral trauma benefits tremendously from a one-on-one relationship with someone outside the friend-and-family circle.

In a therapeutic relationship, the therapist and client become a working team, both committed to the client in a trusting, truthful, constant, and dependable way.

The goal is to work through the emotional suffering, overcome the obstacles, and get from the point of hopelessness to a point of hopefulness. It's building up confidence to face what's on the table.

Were one to try to achieve this with a friend, it could certainly exhaust the friendship. Were one to try to achieve this with a spouse, the load on the spouse could prove overwhelming.

I don't think I could have picked a better therapist than Dr. Sidney Smith to see me through my own hard times. He taught me how to let go of the old self that was no longer there (to stop saying, "I used to be able to…") and to accept – and develop – my new self.

For six years before he went into private practice, Sidney had worked at a hospital with trauma patients. Before he became a psychologist, he had been a priest. I appreciated the spiritual aspect he brought to the "couch." Over the course of our sessions, Sidney encouraged me to renew my relationship with God. Despite the fact that I was Jewish, I decided that I would read sections from Norman Vincent Peale's "The Amazing Power of Positive Thinking" every morning, as a way of finding meaning that would give me strength to get through the day. Even now, I'll return to it when I find that my emotional energy level needs a boost.

Sidney once told me, "Don't draw assumptions from what you fear. Draw assumptions from what you long for."

That made a tremendous difference to me.

In my dissertation, I thanked him for teaching me that one's greatest strength begins at one's broken place.

The Research

I knew what had worked for children with severe learning disabilities. And I knew what had worked for me as a stroke survivor. But I wasn't exactly sure why. Although my interest in brain development was sparked by my own recovery, it was through the research of others that I began to come up with some of the answers. I began to understand how the brain can restore itself – and will restore itself – if presented with the right tools.

As far back as 1874, Charles Darwin noted that the brains of rabbits living in the wild were larger than those of domesticated rabbits. He theorized that wild rabbits had to use their brain more to develop survival strategies.

Seventy-five years later, Donald O. Hebb, a behavioral scientist at McGill University in Montreal, Canada, decided to bring home a few of the rats from a laboratory litter and give them to his children as pets. He encouraged his children to fill the rats' cage with toys and games, and play with their new pets outside the cage.

Later, when he compared the house-pet rats with the laboratory rats on maze-learning abilities, he found that the house-pet rats, who lived in a stimulating and active environment, were cognitively more alert, performed significantly better at maze activities, and were better problem-solvers than their non-stimulated litter mates.

From the 1960s to the 1980s, research scientists at the University of California/Berkeley (David Krech, Mark Rosenzweig, Michael Renner, Marion Diamond, James Connor, and others), worked with rats in cognitively-enriched environments in an attempt to stimulate brain growth and development.

They put a group of rats into an enriched life setting, and compared the group to those groups that remained in standard, unstimulating laboratory conditions. They found that the stimulated group developed a thicker cerebral cortex (the area where higher thinking and problem-solving takes place), and the length and density of the nerve cell dendrites (the branches extending from the neurons that carry messages to the next neuron) were greater.

This same group studied rats that were about two-and-a-half years old (very old by human standards). These rats were given constant support and stimulation, then compared to a control group housed in isolation. The stimulated rats demonstrated significantly enhanced brain adaptation for new experiences and increased cortical growth. According to the researchers, this study challenged the negative myths regarding the aging brain and demonstrated a restorative potential for aging cortical cells.

The research of the 1990s dispelled the negative myths of yesteryear: That once animals – or people – reach adulthood, they may lose brain cells, but they can never grow new ones.

Through research studies at Princeton University in Princeton, New Jersey, Rockefeller University in New York, and the Salk Institute for Biological Studies in La Jolla, California, neurobiologists have found that mice and monkeys – and, in studies conducted by the Salk Institute, humans – are constantly producing new brain cells in the hippocampus, an area of the brain used for forming long-term memories, and in the cortex. (In fact, the study showed, they produce thousands every day.)

In October 1999, the journal, Science, reported on the findings of Elizabeth Gould and Charles G. Gross, two research biologists, at Princeton University, who challenged the long-standing belief that adults never generate new brain cells.

Using macaque monkeys, the two researchers found that thousands of freshly-born neurons arrive each day in three areas of the cerebral cortex where memories are known to be stored – the frontal cortex that is used for decision-making, and two areas on the side of the brain that are used for visual recognition.

The research also showed that mental exercises promoted the growth of new neurons and that mental tasks could double the number and stimulate the growth and development of new neurons in the adult brain.

The Program

In 1991, I went to G. Albyn Davis, one of the leading experts and textbook authors in the field of aphasia, and a professor at the University of Massachusetts/Amherst where I was enrolled in the doctoral program. I wanted him to tell me whether it was possible for me to write my dissertation – and if so, how and what skills I needed.

After talking with me for about an hour, he sent me home with an assignment.

"Write down everything you remember about the topic of your dissertation, and come back in a week," he told me.

Even though I labored over the assignment for hours, I returned the following week with only two paragraphs. Another "Boy, am I in bad shape" reminder. I feared the worst as he read those two paragraphs that I had struggled over for days. Imagine my surprise when he told me, "Now, go home and continue."

Our meetings went on for about three months. Each time he spent an hour – sometimes more – with me, helping me figure out the steps I needed to take, until finally he said, "Now I think you need to take this to your chairperson."

Grace Craig was my chairperson and professor of human development at the time. She acted thrilled to see me and tried to engage me in conversation. I struggled to participate. Then I blurted out, "I can't continue with my dissertation."

I'm not sure that that's what I wanted to say; maybe I was anticipating that she would tell me that I couldn't. By saying it first, I was protecting myself from myself. One of a stroke survivor's survival strategies?

But instead, I heard, "Don't be silly. Go home and write. Get this dissertation finished!"

I thought she was crazy. I found out – after I defended my completed dissertation (three-and-a-half years later) – that she had considered her response crazy, too, and had actually experienced deep feelings of guilt for giving me the encouragement to doing something she did not believe was possible.

Line by line, sentence by sentence, paragraph by paragraph, page by page, I challenged my damaged brain to process, connect, and articulate thoughts and information in words and on paper.

As my writing evolved, with the help of Rockie Blunt, a writing coach, I referred back to the curriculum I had developed for learning disabled students and the concepts and theories on cognitive development that were part of my doctoral education. I considered what I had learned, and continued to learn, in my language therapy sessions.

I began examining the research on brain recovery and brain development, and sought input from highly respected authorities in the various fields. Then, I tried to make sense of it in relation to my own recovery that had occurred through professional and self-initiated rehabilitation.

Keeping all of this in mind, I developed a program of brain therapy that, I believed, would help stimulate the brain cells and refill memory banks that have lost pertinent information – from the name of a grandchild to the recall of a home address to the solving of a complicated equation. Everything that's important in a person's life.

After all, without a long- and short-term working memory, people become disconnected from other people, from daily activities, and from themselves.

The Serper Method of Brain Recovery, Regrowth, and Vitality is designed to harness the natural rebuilding processes within the brain by exposing the person to an intellectually-stimulating learning environment. Designed to motivate participation, it incorporates cerebral exercises into one's daily life by immersing the participant in hard thinking about memories, here-and-now awareness, and future planning, as well as providing exercises that focus on memory, recovery, and stability.

Research aside, I think I developed a much better understanding for what happened to my own brain the first time my computer crashed. Oops. There was no way that I could retrieve the files. Yes, they were gone for good. No, I didn't have any back-up files. But, fortunately, the internal workings were still there; I could begin the slow and tedious process of refilling the files.

I created exercises and activities for myself, and I used them every day, twice a day – one hour in the morning and one hour in the evening. It was the only hope I had. There were no alternatives.

The Serper Method is designed to create an intellectually active environment using cognitive/

memory activities that target 14 different cognitive skills:

    Visual interpretation
    Auditory perception
    Kinesthetic skills
    Verbal delivery
    Comprehension
    Short-term memory
    Long-term memory
    Life-coping skills
    Organizational skills
    Socialization/self-worth
    Creativity/expression
    Problem solving
    Spatial relations
    Application skills

These are the skills that every human being uses every day in order to function effectively and efficiently.

The Serper Method is based on a combination of research/teaching/curriculum development.

Like any good teaching tool, it allows people to experience success and empowers them to take control of one aspect of their lives among the many they've lost control of – and at a time when doctors are inevitably saying to them, "There's not a lot that can be done."

Now, there is something that can be done; there's my brainstorming program.

Your brain is crying out, "Feed me; nourish me; I can still work."

Here's your opportunity to "use it," not "lose it." It is, by no means, a quick process. Don't forget; my becoming an "overnight success" took me five years. It required an inordinate amount of patience.

Your patience will be taxed; you will experience frustration. But whenever this happens, just stop and ask yourself: "What's the alternative?"

Using the Program With People in Early Stages of Alzheimer's Disease

Approximately four million people are affected by Alzheimer's disease, and with the aging of the Baby Boomer population, this number is expected to increase significantly in the coming years. When the last of the baby boomers reach retirement age in 2028, it is anticipated that there will be 16 million people affected by Alzheimer's disease.

Research appears to be focused on finding the medication that will make a difference. In the meantime, opportunities to stave off – or even reverse – what is currently considered the inevitable deterioration of brain function from

Alzheimer's disease – are being overlooked.

It makes me think of a Larry King show I saw recently. Four high-profile people told their stories of hopelessness and frustration over the deterioration of loved ones who had been diagnosed with Alzheimer's disease.

They spoke of their attempts to provide comfort at home before the inevitable placement in a care facility. Then, a doctor from the Mayo Clinic talked about the push in the medical and scientific research community to discover "the pill" to fight the disease. But nobody talked about ways to engage non-medically, and on a day-to-day basis, in the battle against Alzheimer's disease.

When I initially designed my program, I did not imagine that I would be using it with people in the early stages of Alzheimer's disease. Then, a friend's husband was diagnosed with Alzheimer's.

For one year, she and I watched Steve decline. Steve had retired from his business; but he continued to go to an office every day. That gave him the opportunity to continue to use his knowledge and expertise, even though his memory functions were deteriorating, and the doctors were warning them, "Don't expect his level of functioning to last."

One day, as I was updating my friend on the progress I was making with my clients who had suffered strokes and other traumatic brain injury, she interrupted me.

"Why don't you try the program with Steve?" she asked me.

I thought for a moment. Obviously, someone in the early stages of Alzheimer's disease would be very challenging. With my other clients, the cerebral damage had already taken place. The brain was considered to be stable and ready to be challenged. But in a person with Alzheimer's disease, the onslaught to, and deterioration of, the brain was considered to be on-going.

Still, I reasoned, if research had shown that an enriched environment stimulates the growth of the cortex and dendrites in mice, why couldn't the same growth and development serve to inhibit the deterioration caused by Alzheimer's disease?

Although Alzheimer's disease is associated with brain cell deterioration and loss of memory, researchers have found that plasticity of memory function (the way in which nerve cells change and adapt themselves to communicate with other nerve cells as they integrate, coordinate, and categorize information) is evident when cognitive training programs are used with Alzheimer's patients.

In a study conducted at a day hospital with mildly to moderately impaired Alzheimer's disease patients, the experimental group that received cognitive rehabilitation over a period of about eight months appeared to have delayed the disease process when compared to the control group (those who did not receive organized cognitive rehabilitation).

A 1998 study compared three groups – an experimental group that received a medication that stimulates the development of acetylcholine (a chemical that fires off messages from one brain cell to another), along with cognitive training; a control group that received the drug treatment only; and a placebo group that received a sugar pill. Results showed that only the experimental group improved significantly on the MMSE (Mini Mental State Examination).

In addition, the studies from Princeton University, that I cited in the Research chapter of this book, found not only that cognitive tasks could double the number and stimulate the learning capacity of new neurons in the adult hippocampus and cortex, but also that it could help existing neurons live longer.

Of course, I realized that using my program with an Alzheimer's disease client, in contrast to a client who had suffered a stroke, or other cerebral trauma, required a different focus. When I used the program with the latter group, I was helping clients refill their memory banks. To use the program with Alzheimer's clients, my goal would be not only to help people refill their memory banks, but also to help people hold onto the information they still have – and acquire new information.

While we wait for the therapeutic pill or the vaccine (as well as the preventative ones) to be discovered for and tested on people who have been diagnosed in the early stages of Alzheimer's, these people can be maintaining the health of their brain function through my program. They can turn from victims to survivors.

That voice that I had acquired during my own battle returned.

"You can do that," it told me.

So, I said to my friend, "Why not?"

I can't honestly say that Steve cottoned to the program right away. He balked at many of the activities. After all, he told me, he had already been to school. He had no interest in ever doing school work again. He didn't like to write (and he knew that writing was one of the daily requisites of my program). He didn't like factual recall; he hated crossword puzzles (another requisite).

I tried to cajole him; it didn't work. Then, I decided to compare what he had to do with what he had always had to do as a successful businessman.

"When you built your business, did you ever have to do things that you hated to do, but knew that you had to do because you wanted to be successful?" I asked him.

"Of course," he responded.

"Well, welcome to your new business," I told him. "It's called 'You.' Your new business is yourself."

Steve was, in layperson's terms, declining – losing some of his cognitive skills. At the end of the first year of his diagnosis, just prior to his involvement in the program, Steve had been tested at a memory disorders clinic. Results had shown a steady decline in memory and cognitive function areas.

After four months of cognitive exercises from my program, Steve was re-tested at the clinic. The decline had stopped.

After 15 months, further testing results showed stability in all areas, and even some cognitive increases in the areas of recall and attentiveness. (Not surprising when you consider the focus of my program.)

Needless to say, Steve's doctors are stymied. Why has he remained stable? How could he improve? Is he actually winning the battle?

Success breeds success, of course. So, the better Steve feels, he says, the more he commits to the program. In the beginning, I required only that he read one newspaper article of interest to him before he left for his office. Now, he says, not only does he read the article, but also, on his way to work, he keeps thinking about the different ways he can describe his feelings and thoughts about it.

"When I do this, it feels like my (brain) dendrites are tingling and jumping," he once told me. "I'm now aware of my possibilities, and I have a program that keeps me working toward them."

When Steve returned from a recent vacation, I asked him if he was ready to get back to the program. He confessed that he did it even while he was away.

"If I don't do it, I feel lethargic, and I stop thinking," he said.

He has also told me that he is acutely aware of the change that has taken place. He said that the more he works on the activities, especially in the morning, the clearer his thinking becomes, and that this clarity of thinking lasts throughout the day. As a result, he is able to focus better, and has a better overall mental attitude.

When I told him that I was writing this book, and wondered if he had a message to readers, this is what he said:

"Tell people that if they believe they can improve, and they have a way to do it, they will."

How the Program Works

Based on my own experiences of recovery, I knew I had to be where the language was, so that I could start patterning behaviors. But, at the same time, I also realized that unless I refilled my memory banks; relearned how to read and write; count and do math computations; and absorb, process, and categorize events, my brain would atrophy toward – and ultimately into – oblivion. Unless I learned how to express words, my life of garbled language would push me into silence.

The Serper Method format combines cognitive learning theories with games, newspapers, movie plots, lectures, concerts, television programs, puzzles, art and craft projects, and writing activities.

Its goal is to mix life's relevant activities with brain therapy, to provide a way to refill the memory banks, and through the process, enable and enhance social interactions and a feeling of self-worth.

One of the key elements to the program's success is that the exercises are purposeful and, as much as possible, relevant to the specific special interests of the participant. The program also attempts to include activities from the participant's – and caregiver's – daily life. In this way, it serves to normalize one's existence, as much as possible, and in a progressive way. As in any learning situation, a person will retain information faster if the subject matter is of personal interest.

Activities can be self-initiated, or proposed and guided by the caregiver. The goal, of course, is for each participant to become increasingly more self-sufficient in the program, and better able to handle social situations. But even at the early stages, it's important to not feel "locked into" the program. Rather, I strongly encourage adapting the program to individual needs. That's why I call it a self-rehabilitation program.

However, there are certain components to the program that should be adhered to. I introduce the newspaper at the earliest opportunity. The reason: It offers the best common denominator for social interaction. Practically everyone looks at the front page of the newspaper – at least to scan the headlines. So, for the program to work most efficiently, it is essential that the participant engage in newspaper-related activities for at least 30 minutes every morning, and puzzles or workbook-related activities every evening for at least 30 minutes. In between, planned activities: Attend a lecture, go to the movies, take an adult education course (with a spouse, a friend). Go where language is happening. Watch television shows like Wheel of Fortune and Jeopardy.

The important message here is: Every day you have the opportunity to get better. And you will.

How to Use the Serper Method for Your Own Brain Recovery, Regrowth, and Vitality

1. Introduction
2. The Morning Newspaper
3. Crossword Puzzles
4. Jigsaw Puzzles
5. The Serper Method Workbooks and Other Workbook Activities
6. "Games People Play"
7. Reading Activities
8. Listening Activities
9. Writing Activities
10. "Electives"
11. Social Interaction Activities

1. Introduction

Welcome to The Serper Method of Brain Recovery, Regrowth, and Vitality. Participating in this program will give you the opportunity to brainstorm your brain cells with memories and life experiences that were once a normal part of your everyday life.

Although I can't promise you magical, instant recovery, I can provide you with ways to replenish and practice intellectual and social skills that have been impaired by illness or accident.

The Serper Method of Brain Recovery, Regrowth, and Vitality involves starting at the beginning – whatever your beginning is at the time – and working your way up the ladder of, yes, brain recovery, regrowth, and vitality.

I have written that people either live up or down to expectations. If the expectations are low, people will live down to them. If expectations are high, people will live up to them. But I have also written that success breeds success. So, there has to be a balance.

If the expectations set are unrealistically high, people won't be able to live up to them, and they will experience failure. In this case, it is better to engage in easier activities with the expectation that the person will succeed at them than try activities that are at a more difficult level, especially at the beginning when one's confidence is probably at its lowest point.

Warning: There is a real tendency (especially when a loved one is involved) to want to select the more difficult activities because it is so hard to face the reality of how much cerebral damage has been sustained.

Remember, also, that progress is built on

repetition. The activities described below are meant to be done until they are mastered. However, as you know, variety is the spice of life. It is often better to spend less time on more activities than more time on less activities. But because The Serper Method is based on a self-rehabilitation model, ultimately only you can be the judge of the actual number of activities that work best for you. And because nothing is stagnant, each day will probably feel different. Be sure to acknowledge and honor those feelings – and choose the length of time and type of activities accordingly.

The activities involved in The Serper Method can – should – be individualized to account for your individual interests, thereby maximizing your ability to succeed. The only non-negotiable commitment I ask of you is that you set aside at least 30 minutes every morning and 30 minutes every afternoon or early evening.

2. The Morning Newspaper

Using a newspaper as a morning activity is one of the most valuable – and essential – components of The Serper Method. There's also a specific way to incorporate a newspaper into the program, based on ability level.

How To Use The Newspaper Every Morning

The following activities will help you develop three abilities:

■ Provide information that will help you refill your memory banks.

■ Help you maintain an awareness of what's going on in your environment.

■ Contribute to the knowledge you need for social and work interactions.

Level 1 (pre-reading):

Have someone read the headlines from the front page of the newspaper (or any section of the paper) to you, or into a tape recorder. Listen to the words as you look at them in the headlines. Then, close your eyes and try to remember what you heard and saw, and repeat them – in your own words, if possible.

Level 2:

Read the headlines on the front page of the newspaper. (It could be the front page of the sports section.) Then, turn the paper over and list as many headlines as you can recall (either verbally, or write them down on a piece of paper).

Repeat the process until you are able to recall many, most, or even all of the headlines.

Level 3:

Read the headlines on the front page of the newspaper. Then, turn the paper over and list as many headlines as you can recall (either verbally, or write them down on a piece of paper).

Repeat the process until you are able to recall all of the headlines.

Level 4:

Select one of the front page newspaper articles that is the most interesting to you. Read it carefully. Then, turn the paper over and list as many facts as you can remember (either verbally, or write it down on a piece of paper).

Level 5:

Select one of the front page newspaper articles that is the most interesting to you. Read it carefully. Then, turn the paper over and list as many facts as you can remember (either verbally, or write it down on a piece of paper).

Repeat the process until you are able to recall

all of the content. Then, using the "Create Your Own Questions" worksheet (see pages 86-87), write down questions about the article. Answer the questions the following day to see how much you remember about the article. (Note: In the beginning, you may have to re-read the article before answering the questions. Before you know it, you'll be able to answer one or two – then all – of the questions without needing to re-read the article first.)

Level 6:

Choose a newspaper article, and white-out a noun or verb in each sentence. Then re-read the article, filling in the blanks. (This is a excellent way to exercise your memory for word retrieval and word substitution.)

An excellent supplement, by the way, is "Mastering Reading and Language Skills With The Newspaper."

The program (your choice of "On the Record" or "Morning Edition") includes three audio cassettes. You'll find it at most bookstores.

Another way to supplement newspaper activities is by watching the news on television. Write down each topic as you watch, or record each topic into a tape recorder. When the news is over, test yourself. Use your notes or play back your tape to check your answers.

Don't forget, every time you listen to a tape or watch/listen to the news on television, then do a related activity, you're exercising your auditory memory.

"Create Your Own Questions"
(for *newspaper activities*)

Directions: Read an article and create a question about each of the first three paragraphs. Set this sheet aside with the newspaper article until tomorrow. Then, read the questions and answer them. Remember: It's not cheating if you need to go back to the article to find the answers. (Use the worksheet on the next page or create your own.)

Name of article: _____

Date of article: _____

Today's date: _____

PARAGRAPH 1:

Question: _____

_____

Answer: _____

_____

_____

PARAGRAPH 2:

Question: _____

_____

Answer: _____

_____

_____

PARAGRAPH 3:

Question: _____

_____

Answer: _____

_____

3. Crossword Puzzles

Crossword puzzles are part of The Serper Method for three reasons:
- They're a challenge.
- They're an excellent way to refill your memory banks with information you once knew.
- They're a great way to acquire new information.

You can clip crossword puzzles from newspapers or buy easy crossword puzzle books (three copies of each). You'll also find crossword puzzles in The Serper Method workbooks. Or you can – may need to – make your own in order to limit the number of words involved. There's absolutely nothing wrong with a two-word crossword puzzle.

For starters, the two words can be as simple – and relevant – as the names of two of your children or two of your grandchildren.

How To Use Crossword Puzzles Everyday

Like using newspapers every morning, there's a specific way to use crossword puzzles as part of The Serper Method. It covers a three-day period and requires three copies of each crossword puzzle.

Day 1:

Use the first copy and read a question. If you don't know the answer, look it up on the answer page (this is NOT cheating; this is a learning experience), then fill it in on the puzzle.

Repeat the process until you have completed the puzzle.

Day 2:

Use the second blank copy of the same puzzle on the second day, and follow the same procedure.

Day 3:

Use the third blank copy of the same puzzle, and follow the same procedure.

Now, compare how much more you can do on the third day than the first or second days – and give yourself a pat on the back.

4. Jigsaw Puzzles

Whether you start with a 10-piece, a 20-piece, or a 70-piece jigsaw puzzle, the first thing you must do is make room for it on a table that you – and others – pass by frequently, and every time you go by, put a couple of pieces of the puzzle together. Encourage others to participate, too. It's fun to make this a "group" activity.

Why jigsaw puzzles? Jigsaw puzzles tap into the very same cognitive skills that crossword puzzles tap into. Plus, the beauty of jigsaw puzzles is that you can choose visual content that reflects a person's specific interests. Even the easy puzzles for children offer an excellent selection of themes that are visually relevant to an adult. And a "must-have" (though perhaps not immediately) is Milton Bradley's Map of the United States jigsaw puzzle with the World Map on the reverse side.

If you really want to tap into specific interests – and fond memories – you can make your own puzzles by enlarging photographs (12" by 16" enlargements are readily available from any neighborhood photo developing shop) of familiar faces (yes, photos of grandchildren are great ones), locations and faces (you in front of the Eiffel Tower, for example), and/or special events (perhaps a wedding photograph).

All it takes is pasting the photograph onto sturdy cardboard or poster board and cutting it into puzzle-like pieces. (Yet another advantage of creating your own jigsaw puzzle is that you can cut it into as few as two or three pieces.)

5. The Serper Method Workbooks and Other Workbook Activities

You may be wondering about the usefulness of workbooks. After all, when you think back to your school days, who ever liked workbooks? Wasn't that what your teacher gave you for "busy work?" Or "extra" homework?

Still, whether or not you want to admit it, workbooks were – still are – filled with some of the most practical and purposeful skill-building information required for life's mastery. Another advantage of workbooks is that they focus on levels of knowledge. If you're wondering, "How will I ever re-learn everything I need to know?" the answers can be found in The Serper Method workbooks (Levels 1 to 4) and supplemental workbooks that you can purchase in bookstores. For example, Frank Schaffer "Homework Helpers" are especially beneficial at the lowest levels, and include:

- Dot-To-Dot books
- Word Searches (great for visual learning)
- Kindergarten Vocabulary Development
  (basic vocabulary has to come from somewhere)

Another useful workbook series that extends from grades 1 to 8 is the McGraw Hill Learning Materials Spectrum series.

(See sample pages of The Serper Method Workbooks in Appendix A and an order form in Appendix C.)

6. "Games People Play"

Board games are an integral part of the program and are readily available at toy stores – or in your grandchild's toy chest.

Even some of the simplest games (or your creatively simple adaptations of harder games) are surprisingly fun to play. It can be great to feel like a kid again!

■ POOH MEMORY GAME

The *Pooh Memory Game* is an excellent game to exercise your memory – and to play with a young grandchild.

■ SCRABBLE

Don't stop playing *Scrabble* just because you can only come up with two-letter words. Before you know it, your brain will be ready for some three-letter words.

■ BOGGLE

Many games made my time alone go by faster. You'd be surprised at how many of them can be played alone. *Boggle* was one of my favorites. Of course, when you play a game alone, you're always the winner!

■ TRIVIAL PURSUIT

Always think about how to adapt board games to meet your needs. *Trivial Pursuit* (the generic game and/or versions that tap into special interests) doesn't have to actually be played as a game; you can just read the questions and the answers. Then, go back over the cards and see how many answers you can recall. This can be done alone (I used to keep a stack of the cards next to my bed) or with someone else.

■ BATTLESHIP

Games that can be played by two or more players offer a wonderful interactive and social opportunity for the person and his or her caregiver, family, and/or friends. It's also an excellent opportunity for non-contrived verbal interaction. One of my favorite board games for this purpose was – and still is – *Battleship.* Imagine getting to sink all your opponents' ships!

■ CROSSWORDS FOR DUMMIES

Crosswords for Dummies is an excellent crossword puzzle activity supplement.

■ OTHER BOARD GAMES

Here's a sampling of some of the other board games that I used successfully during my own recovery and have used with, or recommended to, my clients.

■ OPERATION SKILL GAME
■ LABYRINTH
■ MAGICAL MAZE

- **CROSSWORDS FOR DUMMIES**
- **UP FOR GRABS**
- **CLUE or CLUE, JR.**

Don't forget, there are travel versions of many of these games. They're usually less expensive than the full-size versions, and they're certainly space-savers.

- **FLASH CARDS**

Flash Cards are excellent for playing matching (*Concentration*) games that can be played alone or with others. (You can also use a deck of cards.) At its simplest, it's a matter of matching two of the same items (e.g., the photograph of a grandchild with the same photograph, or two of the same numbers). Then, progress to matching photograph with name or addition fact with its answer.

Start out with a manageable number of pairs. Then, continue to challenge yourself by increasing the number of pairs. Remember, no matter how few or how many you try, it's still helping you to refill your memory bank.

You can buy all types of flash cards in toy stores – number flashcards, addition, subtraction, multiplication, and division facts flash cards, and sight vocabulary, vowels, and consonants flash cards.

You can – should – also make your own flash card game. Using photographs is, once again, the way to go. A photograph of a grandchild on one side, the name of the grandchild on the flip side. A photograph of the Eiffel Tower on one side, "Eiffel Tower" (or if you want to make it more difficult, "Paris") written on the flip side.

7. Reading Activities

The message here is: Read, read, read. No matter what level you're reading on.

Browse through the Children's (including "Young Adults") section in your local bookstore. You'll probably be surprised at what you'll find.

I'm a big fan of The "STEP into Reading" series. The Step 4 books (for grade 2 to 4 reading levels) offer subject matter that's perfectly suitable for adult tastes. There are biographies of sports figures from the past (Ty Cobb, Jackie Robinson) and the present (Tiger Woods) and biographies of famous political figures. There are also accounts of interesting events (the story of the Vietnam

Veterans Memorial; climbing the world's highest mountain).

For history buffs, I strongly recommend "The Civil War" by Alden R. Carter (as well as his other books about war) and the Cornerstones of Freedom series (my favorite: "The Titanic" by Deborah Kent). All of these books, by the way, have excellent illustrations and photographs.

I also recommend, "Stuck on the U.S.A.: Fascinating Facts about the 50 States."

And, for a well-rounded brain refill experience at a slightly higher (grades 4 to 6) level, there's the "Everything You Need to Know About..." series that includes American History, World History, English, Geography, Math, and Science.

If you find that you have to begin at the lowest level, the Eyewitness Readers series offers outstanding reading materials. On the pre-reading to first grade level, there's "Truck Trouble." (Anyone who has ever driven will enjoy this one.) On the grades 1 – 3 level, there's "Bugs! Bugs! Bugs!" – a great book to read out loud to the grandkids when they come over.

(To the caregiver: If necessary, you can read the story into a tape recorder, and let the person listen while following along in the book. By the way, you can also do this with magazine articles.)

8. Listening Activities

Don't overlook audio-cassettes when you're shopping for books. (You can listen to them at home. Or, how about when you're traveling to the doctor or waiting in the doctor's office?)

Some of my personal favorites are "Lives of the Artists," "Lives of the Presidents," and others from the "Lives of…" series.

I also like "A Children's Book of Heroes." (They're all heroes to adults too, so don't worry about the title.)

And don't forget the self-help and motivational tapes. Tony Robbins' program, "Unlimited Power," is an excellent reminder of why you want to succeed.

How to Use The Serper Method/Listening

And then there are the tapes simply for listening enjoyment. Like, "The 60 Greatest Old Time Radio Shows of the 20th Century" – 30 hours worth of tapes, and many hours of "laugh therapy."

There are also invaluable language and communication development tapes that are designed for people who are learning English for the first time. Well, so are you – again. You'll find them in the Language Reference section of your bookstore, including: "Living Language (Random House), "Practice and Improve Your English" (Passport Books), "American English Pronunciation," and "Listening to Communicate in English" (NTC Publications).

9. Writing Activities

My written language slowly returned, but only when I started working on my doctoral dissertation. No, I'm not suggesting that you write a dissertation – unless you really want to. In the beginning, signing your name to a birthday card or writing "I love you" on a piece of paper and giving it to your spouse are two ways to get your writing skills up and running again. If you're not ready for that yet, then try tracing letters. Book and toy stores carry manuscript and cursive writing books that are excellent starters. There are also the "Learn to Write Numbers," "Learn to Print," and "Learn Handwriting" series that have wipe-off pages, so that you can practice over and over again – and save a tree.

Use a computer, if you have one, but don't stop writing the "old-fashioned" way.

Look through photo albums and write about the people or the places in the photographs. Think back to all the people who have had a positive – and even a negative – impact on your life (remember your first grade teacher?) and write about your memories.

Write letters to others. Write notes to yourself. Write lists. Anything from a grocery list to a list of good advice. One of my most debilitated clients wrote – and illustrated – a children's book and gave it to his seven-year-old son.

As soon as possible, start a daily journal. It doesn't matter what you write in it – or how much you write. It matters that you write in it everyday. By the way, using a hand-held thesaurus/speller can be an invaluable aid.

10. "Electives"

Consider this category the frosting on the cake. It's a time to be at your most creative.

One of my clients loves music and, before her stroke, she had played the flute. I bought a recorder for her, one for her husband (who is also her caregiver), and a copy of "Recorder Fun – Songs for Kids" (Leonard Publishing Co.). Because the songs were so simple, her husband was able to teach himself how to read the notes in the songbook. My client wasn't able to read the music, but she was able to mimic where her husband placed his fingers. He told me that their daily "musicales" provided both of them with some of their happiest moments.

Don't be afraid to try something new. After all, you're a new person. You may not be ready to take an art course – at least not yet, so buy a "How-To" art book. Check out the "I Can Draw…" series. It may have been written for kids, but who says adults don't want to learn how to draw Monsters, Faces, or Comics and Cartoons?

11. Social Interaction Activities

When you commit to The Serper Method of Brain Recovery, Regrowth, and Vitality, you're committing to more than just staying home and working on brain enhancement activities. The primary purpose of the brain enhancement activities is to prepare you for social interaction.

When you read the newspaper every morning and remember the headlines or the content of a news story, you're empowering yourself with information that you can share with others.

When you look over photographs of exciting places you've been, you're re-acquainting yourself with information that you can share when others talk about their travels.

In the beginning, I believed that my own language and thinking losses rendered me unacceptable to family and friends. With the loss of language came the loss of my social self-confidence. As a result, I felt more comfortable staying home and feeling lonely than going out (or inviting someone over) and feeling inadequate. If it weren't for the people who provided me with the necessary social strategies and the friends and family who provided me with the social venues, I might still be home alone.

Looking back, I realize that it took three things to fortify myself for social situations: courage, preparation, and practice. If you work on mastering these three components, the exercises below will soon become part of your social repertoire.

Level 1:

Write down – or have someone else write down – what you want to say. It can be as simple as "How are you?" or "It's good to see you."

If you cannot read or pronounce the words,

have someone else say them to you; then, you repeat them. Even better, have someone tape the words (pausing between words, sentences, or phrases), so that you can listen and repeat.

Level 2:

Practice asking questions – the kind of questions that keep other people talking about themselves.

Practice being an active listener. Even if you don't understand what the person is saying, stay focused and interested(-appearing) by making eye contact and intermittently nodding your head. Pay attention to the facial expressions of the talker. Then replicate them.

Level 3:

Before you go to a small gathering, party, or event, think about the people you expect to be there. Then, write down their names (or have someone else write them down for you) and practice saying them. (You might want to use a tape recorder.)

Write down and rehearse what you know

about these people – where they live, what they do for a living, what they do for pleasure, how many children they have, where they've traveled, what their hobbies are, etc. Then, write down questions you could ask, and practice asking them. For example:

"How are your children? Where are they living? What are they doing?"

"How is your skiing (golf, tennis)?"

"Take any trips recently? How was the weather?"

It's a good idea to tape yourself asking these questions, so that you can listen to/master the proper voice inflections.

(Note: You can also use the Social/Work Planner worksheets on pages 118-120.)

Here's another tip: Bring your notes with you in your pocket or purse. If necessary, review them in the privacy of a bathroom stall. After all, preparation can be done in any place at any time.

Level 4:

Put yourself out there. Attend lectures and

concerts. Sign up for an adult education class. Find a music teacher who specializes in teaching adults how to play an instrument. (Haven't you always wanted to play the piano? Or drums?) If you can learn English again, how about learning Spanish?

And remember, no matter how frustrated you may feel, don't give up. Every brain must be stoked and fired if it is to become – and remain – strong and vibrant. Your brain has been injured. Now, it must be challenged to regain its memory and vitality. Today, you are beginning the process of once again becoming responsible for the rehabilitation of your brain power. Like any other overnight success story, it's going to take time.

So, here's something to keep in mind:

DROP

The key to The Serper Method of
Brain Recovery, Regrowth, and Vitality:
Determination+Resiliency+Optimism+Perserverance=
DROP EVERYTHING.
(YOU'VE GOT A JOB TO DO.)

Social/Work Planner

Fill in the following information BEFORE your social or work engagement:

1. Where am I going? _____
_____
_____

2. Why am I going there? _____
_____
_____

3. Who'll be there?   What they do?   What they like?

_____   _____   _____
_____   _____   _____
_____   _____   _____
_____   _____   _____

4. What topics will I talk or ask questions* about? And to whom?

*Examples of questions: How are your children? Where are they living? What are they doing? How is your skiing (golf, tennis)? Take any trips recently? How was the weather?

Name of person _____

Questions _____

_____

_____

Name of person _____

Questions _____

_____

_____

Name of person _____

Questions _____

_____

_____

Name of person _____

Questions _____

_____

_____

Reminder: Nod your head and listen with interest when the person responds to your questions. Another reminder: Don't forget to bring this completed form with you in case you need to refer to it.

Fill in the following information AFTER your social or work engagement:

1. Where did I go? _____
_____

2. Who was there? _____
_____
_____

3. What I thought of the experience? _____
_____
_____
_____

4. Why? _____
_____
_____
_____

APPENDIX A

1. The Serper Method Workbook Sample (Level 2 Math)
2. The Serper Method Workbook Sample (Level 2 Reading)

Appendix A

1. The Serper Method Workbook Sample (Level 2 Math)

The most important math skills that an adult needs to recover involve time and money. Because the learner can actually handle the money, the activity is more concrete and easier to master, so make sure that when you're doing these problems, you have coins and bills handy. (Don't worry, there's nothing that involves more than a $20 bill.)

Use a clock to help with the time problems. (If you don't want to use a real clock, you can find toy clocks in most toy stores.)

Appendix A

Word problems: AT THE MOVIES

1. Regular admission costs $7 at the General Cinema; admission for senior citizens at least 60 years old and children 10 or younger is $3.50. How much will it cost you to go to a movie?

2. How much less does it cost a senior citizen or child to go to the General Cinema?

3. John is 65; his wife is 60. How much will it cost them to go to General Cinema?

4. 35-year-old Nancy is going to take her 13-year-old daughter and 9-year-old son to the General Cinema. How much money is she going to need for the three of them? _____

5. Nancy only has a $20 bill. How much change will she get back?_____

6. What can she spend it on?
Popcorn: $4.75 (Yes? No?) M&Ms: $2.25 (Yes? No?)
Diet Coke: $2.50 (Yes? No?)

Appendix A

7. How much money would she need if she wanted to buy the popcorn, the candy, and the drink?

8. How much more money would she need besides the change she got from the $20?

9. The movie that Nancy wants to see is 2 hours. The movie her kids want to see is 2 hours, 10 minutes. How long will Nancy have to wait for her kids after her movie gets out?

10. The movie starts at 4:00 p.m. and gets out at 5:55 p.m. How long does the movie last?

Answers: 1. Depends on person's age.
2. $3.50
3. $7.00
4. $17.50
5. $2.50
6. No; yes; yes
7. $9.50
8. $7.00
9. 10 minutes
10. 1 hour, 55 minutes

Appendix A

2. The Serper Method Workbook Sample (Level 2 Reading)

Directions: Read this short story, then answer the questions.

(Note to caregivers: Questions can be answered verbally at first and then in writing on a separate piece of paper. They can also be answered by looking back at the text at first and then answered from memory.)

ANNA ELEANOR ROOSEVELT

Eleanor Roosevelt was born on October 11, 1884 into one of New York's richest families. Her first name was Anna, but everyone called her Eleanor. She was not good looking, and her mother used to tell her, "You have no looks, so see to it that you have manners."

And so she did. She was also very bright and wanted to become a teacher, but in those days wealthy women were expected to marry well, and at a young age.

By the time she was 19 years old, Franklin Delano Roosevelt, one of Eleanor's distant cousins, had proposed to her. And she had accepted.

Questions:

1. Where was Eleanor Roosevelt born?

_____

2. What was her real first name?

_____

Appendix A

3. How old was she when Franklin Roosevelt proposed to her?

_____

4. Do you think she wanted to get married?_____
Why?

_____

_____

_____

5. Writing Assignment (Level 1):
Look over the story again; then write down everything you remember.

   Writing Assignment (Level 2):
Without looking over the story again, write down everything you remember.

   Writing Assignment (Level 3):
Write about a woman whom you admire. (Tell about the qualities you most admire and why.)

APPENDIX B
Self-Help Books for Caregivers

From Panic to Power by Lucinda Bassett (HarperCollins)

Honoring the Self by Nathaniel Branden (Bantam Books)

Taking Responsibility by Nathaniel Branden (Simon & Schuster)

When the Going Gets Tough, the Tough Lighten Up by Terry Braverman (Mental Floss Publications)

Stop Worrying by Frank Bruno, PhD (MacMillan)

Make the Most of your Mind by Tony Buzan (Simon & Schuster)

Chicken Soup for the Soul by Jack Canfield and Mark Victor Hansen (Health Communications)

The Stress Management Source Book by J. Barton Cunningham, PhD (Lowell House)

The Soul's Companion by Tian Dayton, PhD (Health Communications)

Writing as a Way of Healing by Louise De Salvo, PhD (Harper San Francisco)

Forgiving Yourself by Beverly Flanigan (MacMillan)

Woulda, Coulda, Shoulda by Dr. Arthur Freeman and Rose DeWolf (Harper Perennial)

Are You in Control by Wendy Grant (Element)

Making Stress Work for You by Helen Graham (The Crossing Press)

Emotional First Aid by Sean Haldane (Station Hill)

What to Say When You Talk to Your Self by Shad Helmstetter, PhD (Pocket Books)

So, Stick a Geranium in Your Hat and Be Happy by Barbara Johnson (Word Publishing)

Wherever You Go, There You Are by Jon Kabat-Zinn (Hyperion)

Bringing Out the Best in People by Alan Loy McGinnis (Angsburg)

The Daily Relaxer by Matthew McKay, PhD and Patrick Fanning (New Harbinger Publication)

The Amazing Power of Positive Thinking by Norman Vincent Peale (Ballantine Books)

Living Through Personal Crisis by Ann Kaiser Stearns (Ballantine)

A Gift of Hope: How We Survive Our Tragedies by Robert L. Veninga (Ballantine)

The Resilient Spirit by Polly Young-Eisendrath (Addison-Wesley)

The following are recommended Feldenkrais Method books:

Awareness Through Movement by Moishe Feldenkrais (Harper San Francisco)

Awareness Heals by Steven Shafarman (Addison Wesley)

Relaxercise by David Zeniach-Bersia, Kaethe Zeniach-Bersia, and Mark Reese (Harper San Francisco)

APPENDIX C:
Book and Workbook Order Forms

Appendix C

BOOK ORDER FORM

To order additional copies of *Brainstorming: The Serper Method of Brain Recovery, Regrowth, and Vitality*, fill out the information below and mail to:

**Brain Enhancement Services, Inc.
770 Boylston Street, Suite 17-I
Boston, MA 02199
(Attn: Book order)
Or you can order by phone with a MasterCard or Visa by calling: 800-240-3778.**

Please send _____ copies of *Brainstorming: The Serper Method of Brain Recovery, Regrowth, and Vitality* at $14.95 per book + $3.95 for shipping and handling per book to:

Name: _____

Address: _____

City: _____ State: _____ Zip: _____

Phone: _____

Make checks payable to: Brain Enhancement Services, Inc.

If you are paying with a credit card:

MasterCard: _____ exp. date: _____

Visa: _____ exp. date: _____

Appendix C

WORKBOOK ORDER FORM

To order *Brainstorming: The Serper Method of Brain Recovery, Regrowth, and Vitality* WORKBOOKS fill out the information below and mail to:

    Brain Enhancement Services, Inc.
    770 Boylston Street, Suite 17-I
    Boston, MA 02199
    (Attn: Workbook order)

Or you can order by phone with a MasterCard or Visa by calling: 800-240-3778.

Check the workbook(s) you wish to order:
☐ Level 1   ☐ Level 2   ☐ Level 3   ☐ Level 4
at $9.95 per book + $3.95 for shipping and handling.

Name: _____

Address: _____

City: _____ State: _____ Zip: _____

Phone: _____

Make checks payable to: Brain Enhancement Services, Inc.

If you are paying with a credit card:

MasterCard:_____ exp. date:_____

Visa: _____ exp. date:_____

To learn more about
Brain Enhancement Services, Inc.,
visit us on the web at:
www.brainenhance.com